S

GW00691790

QUESTIONS & ANSWERS

FOR

SO CALLED EXPERTS

BY

AMANDA SCOTT

IDEAS UNLIMITED (PUBLISHING)

Published by:
Ideas Unlimited (Publishing)
P.O. Box 125, Portsmouth
Hampshire PO1 4PP

© **1995 Ideas Unlimited (Publishing) & Amanda Scott**

ISBN: 1 871964 172

Printed & Bound in Great Britain.

SOME USEFUL UK ADDRESSES

These are mainly head offices (correct at time of going to press)

Beaumont Society
BM Box 3084
London WC1N 3XX
(Advice for transvestites)

British Pregnancy Advisory Service
Austy Manor
Wootton Wawen
West Midlands
01564 793225

Gay Youth Movement
BM Gym
London WC1N 3XX
0171 317 9690

Health Education Authority
78 New Oxford Street
London WC1 1AH
0171 631 0930

Institute of Psychosexual Medicine
11 Chandos Street
London W1M 9DE
0171 580 0631

London Lesbian & Gay Switchboard
BM Switchboard
London WC1N 3XX
0171 837 7324

Rape Crisis Centre
PO Box 69
London WC1X 9NJ
0171 916 5466

Sexual Problems of the Disabled
286 Camden Road
London N7 OBT
0171 607 8851

Terrence Higgins Trust
52 - 54 Grays Inn Road
London WC1X 8JU
0171 242 1010.

The Family Planning Association
27 - 35 Mortimer Street
London W1N 7RJ
0171 636 0366

Women's Health & Reproductive
Rights Centre
52 - 54 Featherstone Street
London EC1Y 8RT
0171 251 6332

ACKNOWLEGDEMENTS

Bluff Your Way In Sex (Tim Webb/Sarah Brewer) Ravette Books.

Contraception - The Facts (Peter Bromwich/Tony Parsons)
Oxford Medical.

Gray's Anatomy Churchill Livingstone.

Infertility (Prof. Robert Winston) Optima.

Law - A Modern Introduction (Paul Denham) Hoder & Stoughton.

Patterns Of Sexual Behaviour (CS Ford) Methuen

Safe Sex (Dr Elliot Philipp) Columbus Books.

The Adolescent Years (Pat Petrie) Michael Joseph.

The Facts About Child Sexual Abuse (Bill Gillham) Cassell.

Women & The Aids Crisis (Diane Richardson) Pandora.

Women's Health (Sandra Cabot) Pan Books.

Your Sex Life (Peter Bromwich) Harrap.

Jean Hurst : Terrence Higgins Trust.

Marion Cooper Advisory Service : Smith & Nephew

Nigel Hill : London School of Hygiene and Tropical Medicine.

INTRODUCTION

As we all know, sex has been around for a long time. Everyone likes to think they're experts on the subject but, in reality, this is far from the truth. There are a lot of questions that many of us are too shy or too embarrassed to ask.

SEX: QUESTIONS AND ANSWERS takes an amusing look at a subject that is close to all our hearts - and bodies! The questions were sent in by ordinary people of all ages and from all walks of life. They range from more direct questions to the more unusual.

The questions don't appear in any specific order but have been answered as factually as possible and at random.

We know you'll enjoy this book and we hope to include, in our next edition, more questions together with light-hearted stories sent in by readers. Topics like 'My first sexual experience' or 'When I was on holiday...' should provide some very amusing reading. Don't worry, you can write anonymously. No names and addresses will be printed ... unless, of course, you want to see your name in print!

Ah well, on with the questions ... or more to the point, on with the answers!

AMANDA SCOTT

1. When was the first condom invented or discovered?

The first one I 'discovered' was lying in a puddle behind the bike sheds at my primary school!

Condoms, rubber johnnies, French letters or, as the French say, capotes Anglais, (an English cloak or cape) have been around a long time. As far as we know, five hundred years ago Gabriel Fallopius, an Italian, invented a linen sheath which was treated with chemicals. It covered the top half of the penis and was meant to act not only as a contraceptive but also to protect against venereal disease. Apparently it was thick and awkward to use but was a real step forward.

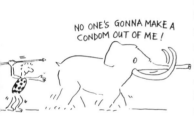

NO ONE'S GONNA MAKE A CONDOM OUT OF ME !

However, condoms were probably around in Egyptian times. Condom devices appear in cave paintings in France and a fish-skin condom was found down a 13th century well in Wales. The Chinese had linen and leather condoms... but the truth is, we simply don't know the exact origin.

A Frenchman, the Marquis de Sevigne, made a membrane from a cow's intestines and in Charles II's time, Dr Condom 'invented' the condom from pig's bladders and sheep's intestines. No doubt a little trial and error was needed until he got the correct age of the correct animal just right!

2. Can I become pregnant while I am having my period?

The only sure way of not geting pregnant at any time is by keeping your panties on, your legs tightly crossed and staying away from the opposite sex!

You can become pregnant during your period and at all other times in your monthly cycle, particularly during the middle of the month when you are ovulating. All women, are different and some are more likely to become pregnant at varying times. After all, Nature is very clever and is <u>responsible</u> for ensuring the human race continues... no matter what.

Should you not wish to become pregnant, it's best not to take chances. There are many forms of contraception available... some are mentioned later in this book. Remember, a single sperm doesn't like to take no for an answer.

Did you know: With hi-tech blood screening, the chance of contracting the Aids virus in a blood transfusion in Britain is one in one million.

Did you know: Humans grow more hair, per square centimetre, than chimpanzees.

Did you know: In 1994, the average age for couples having their first child was 28 years. In 1971, it was just over 23.5 years.

3. My vagina nearly always makes strange 'farting' noises during or just after intercourse. How can I prevent this from happening?

Are you sure it's your front passage that's making all the noise? Sometimes women who perform yoga, that is relaxing and standing on their heads, find that air is drawn into the vagina and consequently it makes an embarrassing noise when they stand upright again. You must stop making love while standing on your head!

Seriously, this trapped air in the vagina is quite common and is caused by slight looseness in the vaginal passage. During sexual arousal and intercourse the vagina tends to enlarge and the walls expand. Your partner's penis

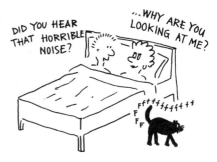

forces air in by his pumping actions and it becomes compressed air. Eventually it makes a noise when it comes out. It's all his fault! Special floor exercises (Kegal Exercises) may strengthen the vaginal muscles but, meanwhile, just try to laugh it off.

Did you know: In Romania, before the 1989 revolution, contraception and abortion were banned and there was an obligation for couples to have at least five children.

4. Why do some couples make a lot of noise when they make love?

How do you know? You haven't had that glass against the wall again, have you?

Sex can be a noisy business. Some couples make a lot of grunting, groaning, sighing and screaming noises. Some just like showing off. It all depends on temperament and passion. Some create an 'atmosphere', and some make a noise simply to drown out the noise of the bedsprings!

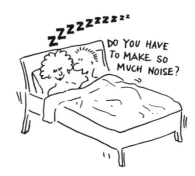

Television and movies nearly always show noisy sex scenes (it's funny that most directors and producers are men)! These scenes have almost become a cliché devised by the film director because that's what they believe the viewing audience wants and expects. All that noise certainly keeps viewers watching, but I'm always trying to see where they pin the hidden microphone!

> Did you know: Chimpanzees have a very promiscuous mating system and have nine times the sperm count of a gorilla.

5. What is the most contagious sexually transmitted disease (STD) known?

'Crabs' are very contagious - you can almost catch them by just thinking about sex! The chance of getting pediculosis pubis, or crabs, from one sexual exposure (with an infected partner) is over 90 percent! The pubic louse is an ugly little creature with six strong, long hairy legs which enable it to cling on to pubic hair. However, they can be found on all hairy parts - even the eyelids, but pubic lice are different from head lice.

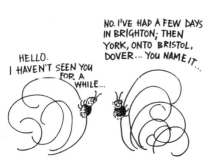

Crabs cannot be caught from toilet seats but can be acquired from dirty, infected bedclothes etc. They cause itching and inflammation due to scratching and their blood-sucking way of life. They are rarely serious and can be easily got rid of - no, not by using a large hammer - but by an insecticidal shampoo.

Did you know: In a study of unfaithful men and women, it took 5.2 years of marriage for men and 4.5 years of marriage for women to become unfaithful.

6. I've heard of men with really large penises... and I want one! Is there any way I can have my best friend made bigger?

First of all, how do you know you've got a 'tiddler'? Don't you think you're worrying unnecessarily? After all we know that some men 'think' with their dicks and maybe you ought to consider this possibility.

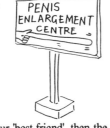

However, according to certain consultant neurologist, there are men with micro-penises where the penis is the size of the first joint of the little finger! If this is the case with your 'best friend'. then the next paragraph might be of real interest. With much opposition from the British Medical Establishment, a Men's Institute for Cosmetic Surgery is about to be opened by a American urologist - a Dr Melvyn Rosenstein. He claims he can lengthen the penis by cutting the suspensery ligament which attaches it to the pubic bone and thereby exposing the penis root. This is then covered by skin from the front of the pubic bone. It all sounds so simple, you could almost do it yourself!

The thickness of the penis can easily be increased by extra fat deposits being implanted by liposuction injection. The operation could add five to eight centimetres to the length and increase the thickness by 50 percent. Normal sexual activity can resume within about a month.

7. My husband feels like sex only once a month, and it's ruining our sex-life. We just haven't got one. What can I do?

Couples make love about two or three times a week depending upon their ages, circumstances and sexual needs.... let's face it, some couples only <u>talk</u> about two or three times a week!

Sometimes there are a lot of underlying factors which can affect a low sex-drive in both sexes. Consequently, there are a lot of questions I would like to ask you before I answer your question. For instance, I don't know your husband's age, his physical condition, his mental condition of how long he has been like this. A

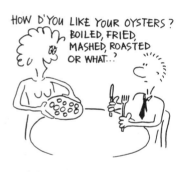

HOW D'YOU LIKE YOUR OYSTERS? BOILED, FRIED, MASHED, ROASTED OR WHAT...?

relationship shift such as an addition to your family can have a direct effect on his emotions. All these things play their part.

Alcohol consumption, stress, obesity, family worries outside the marriage, lack of exercise - all wrapped up with the daily treadmill of life can result in a lack of libido. Maybe he is having an affair. Maybe the problem lies with you! You could be a nagging overweight lump of lard!

8. Do only boys have wet dreams?

A wet dream or 'nocturnal emission' is the involuntary ejaculation of semen in the night. In other words it's like a 'phantom' hand

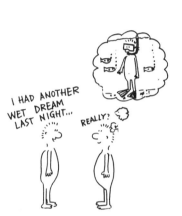

masturbating you. It's quite natural, very common and only happens to males. They usually occur in boys around puberty but can continue for years. It's just Nature's way of making sure everything's working the way it should - a kind of overflow. Adult men even have them.

Wet dreams happen in the night (usually just before waking) and sometimes follow an erotic dream.

Sometimes this dream is forgotten or sometimes a wet dream will just happen! Some adolescents never have them but this doesn't mean they're not making enough sperm or are 'drying up'... it's just the way it is.

Did you know: 0.5 percent of the population, through genetic maldevelopment, should have been born the opposite sex.

Did you know: Woody Allen once said 'Sex is the most fun you can have without laughing'.

9. Will a vasectomy affect my man's libido?

This all depends on whether he has any libido in the first place!

Sterilisation through having a vasectomy is usually permanent and, consequently, men react in different ways. Sometimes men take a little time in getting used to the idea that they've had the 'snip' - even after counselling. A temporary disinterest in sex is quite common.

Some feel guilty that part of their manhood has been 'tampered with' - even though semen, the fluid in which the sperm 'swim' is still produced mainly by the prostate gland and released in the same way when having intercourse. The orgasmic pleasures of having sex are still the same. But, sometimes the guilt feeling stems from a partner railroading the man into having a vasectomy which can lead to all sorts of psychological problems and relationship difficulties.

Some men feel a positive sense of sexual freedom knowing that contraception is no longer necessary. Research indicates that most men feel pleased and some even wish they'd had the operation earlier.

After a vasectomy sperm is still produced by the testes (balls) and some men worry unnecessarily that a huge 'sperm mountain' is building up inside their testicles. Of course this is a myth: like all other unwanted cells in the body, they are simply broken down and their constituents recycled.

10. Why is the end of a penis that funny shape?

Well, we asked over 100 penises and they all agreed they're not funny at all! In fact, they're the perfect shape to get the maximum pleasure out of the sexual act.

Most of the sensitive nerve endings are on the top and the sides of the tip (the glans) which is essential as humans are the only creatures which mate, face to face. The man's forward thrusting ensures that most of the nerve endings are in contact with the vaginal wall at any one time. The foreskin is also important as it can provide some protection against the elements, insects and what-have-you. This has to be connected in some way, so the underneath of the tip seemed the best place. The foreskin is sort of held in place by a thin piece of skin called the prepuce. So, it might appear to look 'funny' but that's because you're not a penis!

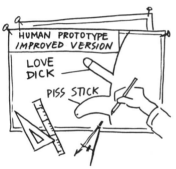

What I want to know is why a penis doubles up as a super-sensitive reproduction organ and a fancy hose-pipe for urine. Someone didn't think the design through properly, I reckon...

11. Why is pubic hair short and curly?

I knew this question would be sent in! If it wasn't short and curly it would hang down to your knees!

According to the Institute of Trichologists, London (who deal with all hair problems) it grows like this because of its short growth cycle and the spiralled nature of the hair follicle that produces it. There is no real reason why it is confined to the pubic area, but it could be for warmth, protection, or for trapping secretions of certain (apocrine) glands. It just grows on the release

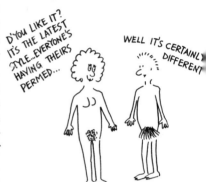

of androgens - or sex hormones, on reaching puberty. It's an axillary type of hair and is different from other types which grow on our bodies.

Pubic hair can differ in colour from our other hair colouring - just like eyebrows or beards are sometimes different colours. Some people don't have any pubic hair. This is a genetic trait or can be caused by disease - a form of Alopecia areata. Itching occurs when the hair starts to grow back on itself and irritates the surrounding skin. Negroes and oriental people tend to have less pubic hair.

So now you know! Don't forget those little crabs!

12. Once and for all, does size really matter?

The erect penis comes in every shape, colour and speed. It's not the length of the penis that counts, it's the thickness, the speed of use, and, above all, the 'arousal factor' of the woman.

After all, the unaroused vagina, is only, on average, 10 cms in length... a little longer when it's aroused. In theory, damage could occur to the cervix (the opening of the womb) if the penis was too long! The 'tightness' of the vagina also plays a part in providing pleasure to both parties because the vaginal walls and the shaft of the penis both have erogenous nerve endings. There are other factors which are important to bear in mind: stress levels, drug/medication, age, the woman's menstrual cycle, stability in the relationship, sexual positions, the time, the place and even alcohol levels. I must point out that the clitoris and the tip of the penis have roughly the same amount of compact nerve endings. Both sexes experience the same kind of pleasure, it's just that sometimes women do not experience a climax in the same way that a man does. Sometimes it's non-existent. Sometimes it's a multi-orgasm... Unfortunately, some men still relate a big penis with ego and manhood. Hands up , how many dick heads do you know?

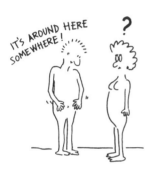

13. My boyfriend ejaculates at the drop of a hat. What can I do to keep him going longer?

He's got a very common condition called 'whippet willie'! Rapid ejaculation in young men is caused by sexual over excitement and even the sensation of rolling a condom on to the penis is enough to bring on an orgasm! It is extremely embarrassing and the young man feels he's not in control of his body, which of course he isn't. Some therapists suggest that any delay in the mechanism is due to a 'disease' of civilisation. However, Neanderthal man needed to ejaculate as soon as possible before being attacked and eaten! It's assumed that we've simply evolved a bit... or in your fella's case - not evolved very much!

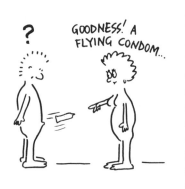

Premature ejaculation is virtually the norm for the sexually inexperienced: there's not much you can do about it. Alcohol may delay things a bit, or he can try thinking about other things as a form of distraction. Sometimes stress can cause overexcitement and sex is a definite release valve. The condition can be brought on as a result of sexual abstinence - the first ejaculation after a period of waiting, will often happen rapidly.

You could say that it's your 'fault'... he finds you too sexy and just can't wait to make love! Try and not to overeact and treat this problem as a non-event: laugh it off in a way that won't damage his self-esteem and his manliness.

After a quarter of an hour or so, he'll be ready for the real thing: try to regard the first orgasm as a rehearsal... you don't have much choice - he can't unejaculate!

Some women try squeezing the tip of the penis a few times when the man feels he's going to come. They count to ten to supress an ejaculation and then repeat the squeezing each time the urge to ejaculate returns! All this sounds a bit dubious to me... you don't often see these going - ons in the movies. I've never seen a steamy love scene where the superstud gets his willie squeezed every 15 seconds!

Some young men realise that this problem is a real problem and when they know they are going to have sexual intercourse they masturbate before hand to suppress the ejaculatory process. Otherwise they just have to grin and bear it!

Did you know: According to the World Health Organisation, 80 million people worldwide would have contracted the AIDS virus by the year 2000.

Did you know: Sperms swim on average at the rate of 18cm (7ins) per hour. It would take one, 2,500 years to swim from New York to Land's End, Cornwall.

14. Why does my wife seem to have so many 'headaches'?

I dunno! Ask her - she may say you're the 'headache'!

Women have headaches two and a half times more than men - on average. These sometimes turn into real 'pounders' called migraine. Anyone who suffers from migraine will know the difference. Accordingly, Dr E Spierings, a top neurologist, says migraine is somewhat hereditary. So, your wife's headaches could be caused by your mother-in-law!

Other trigger factors bring on headaches: stress, weather changes, alcohol, food allergies, fatigue, oral contraceptives, oversleeping, lack of food and, our old favourite, hormones.

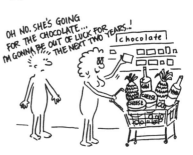

Women experience most headaches in the middle of their monthly cycle and when they're having a period (which doesn't give much time left)!

In a recent survey of migraine sufferers, attacks were brought on by cheese (40%), chocolate (33%), alcohol (23%) and citrus fruits (21%). But the biggest factor of all was stress (44%). Maybe she's stressed because you're mean and don't give her enough love and attention. I knew it was all your fault!

15. I've heard that two lovers can become 'stuck' together during intercourse by a vacuum being created in the vagina and actually 'sucking' the penis in. Is this true?

We've all heard that one... and some people can even name names! No, it's not true.

But, in theory, it could happen if the woman suffered from vaginismus. This condition is caused by the psychological concerns over sex - the vaginal muscles contract so tightly, the man simply can't withdraw his penis.

The eventual subsidence of his erection would make this episode short-lived but his recollection would no doubt be long-lived! (Animals such as foxes, do get 'stuck' together, but that's another answer in another book).

16. What is the longest penis in the world?

Who writes these questions?!

Relative to its size, the barnacle - which is both male and female - has the longest penis in the world. It doesn't have much option really, as it can't move from the underwater spot it calls home. Its penis is a whopper... over 40 times the length of its body! That's like your average man having a dick measuring 75 metres! It would extend over the roof of an average house - and down the other side!

17. I am 18 and my girlfriend is 16.
How can I persuade her to have sex with me?

What is this - wham, bam, thank you ma'm?

You cannot simply pressurise your girlfriend into having intercourse with you just because it suits you. What are you, a man or a monster? We all know that guys of your age think of little else than getting their ends away, but be honest with yourself... do you really respect your girlfriend and understand what she wants? She probably thinks of nothing else but you between her legs - however, any coercing on your behalf is strictly out of order if she's not ready. It could lead to harsh words being spoken and in turn these will lead to a fight. You might end up losing her - perhaps to someone who's prepared to wait, to show her more respect, more understanding, more reassurance and more care that she obviously needs.

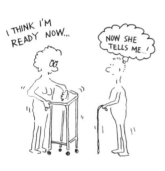

In a few words, she probably needs to be shown more love. It's not simply'... of course I love you - now get 'em off...' That's not love, that's sex. There is a big difference. After all, it doesn't really take too much brainpower for any two people to strip off and get stuck in. But making love is a different item altogether. Of course you're bound to look at things differently, but, if you're a real man, you'll wait until she's ready.

Be patient, be reasonable, be a little less one-sided. Continue with your relationship and don't worry, she'll let you know when she's ready.

18. Why does my vagina sometimes smell fishy?
I keep myself clean but the smell just comes back.

The vagina is the 'tube' which leads from the front of your body to your womb. It's really a long muscle which surrounds a delicate but strong inner lining.

The cells lining the vagina are constantly being replaced to keep you in tip-top condition. Dead cells have nowhere to go and find their way to the front, your vaginal lips. (Sometimes a clear, non-smelly discharge can be felt or seen. This is quite normal. However, this discharge can really smell awful when some women don't keep themselves clean on a regular basis.)

The dead cells that your vagina sheds are constantly being broken down by your vagina's natural defences - a bacteria called lactobacillus. With some women there simply isn't enough lactobacillus to break down all the dead cells so other bacteria move in and cause that fishy smell. Antibiotics can also cause this fishy smell because they're there to kill off bacteria and they kill off your natural lactobacillus as well! You just can't win.

19 I've heard of aphrodisiacs... are there any that really work and, if so, how do they work?

An aphrodisiac is any drug that stimulates sexual desire and performance. In reality one doesn't exist. Scientists over the years have really tried their best and in some countries millions of people really swear by powered rhino horn, liquid incense, animal testes (raw and cooked), ground reindeer antlers, Spanish fly - which is prepared from crushed green blister beetles, turtle eggs, ginseng root and 'potions with a promise'! Not one of these concoctions works... it's all in the mind: a sort of self-induced fantasy. If the person who's taking the aphrodisiac thinks it's going to work, well, it probably will... only in their mind. Even in Europe, the pursuit of this mythical dream goes on: oysters (which contain lethal cadmium) are consumed by the dozen - fortunes are spent on exotic perfumes which contain animal pheromones (none of which trigger irresistible desire in humans), - expensive chocolates can bring on headaches - designer drugs can be addictive while having numerous side-effects by upsetting our delicate hormone balance - but still the search for an aphrodisiac continues.

Tranquillisers, alcohol, and drugs all tend to 'relax' the brain and so we tend to lose our sexual inhibitions. You could say that a romantic film, moonlight, fast cars, sensual music, provocative clothes and exotic locations are mood-altering 'drugs', but the only real aphrodisiac, in the true sense of the word, is the mind.

20. How do lesbians make love?

Women who are gay have a distinct disadvantage. (We're all adults here and we all know what that means!)

Gay women make love in much the same way as heterosexual couples. They like to kiss, hug, rub breasts and bodies together, share sexual fantasies, masturbate together, all-over body kiss, bathe together, suck each other nipples and generally have a good time!

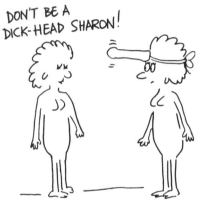

Obviously, contraception is not an issue and so in many ways, lesbians have more sexual freedom than most but their sexual activities can be restricted by their monthly periods. Some lesbians have stable relationships which continue all their lives - and in some states in America gay women can marry. With some couples there may be a dominant partner who prefers to take a more active role in the sexual side of the relationship. She may strap on a dildo, which is penis shaped, and penetrate her partner. But, some couples find using a dildo too masculine - it all depends on the relationship and personal preferences.

21. I want to start getting really intimate with my girlfriend: I don't want to pick the wrong time of the month. How can I tell whether she's having a period without asking her?

There's no real way of telling other than asking her outright - which could be embarrassing for you both. Many girls try to keep the fact that they're having a period a secret. Why should anyone else know? Some girls like to 'compare notes' but it's unusual for girls to discuss such things with their boyfriends ... but times are changing.

If you know her that well, you might be able to detect a few tell-tale signs: her breasts might become tender - so be gentle. She may be slightly moody or irritable or you might get right up her nose for no apparent reason. You may retaliate and think it's something you've said or done - or even something you've not said or not done! She will obviously give you the cold shoulder when you try to get really intimate, so in many ways she'll let you know.

She may not feel like doing too much, in the way of strenuous activity - y'know, heavy partying, swimming, walking miles, horse-riding, that sort of thing.

Once you've determined when her period is, you must reckon on it lasting about three to five days. It's then about 28 days till the next one - so you'd better make the most of it while you can.

22. How do pregnancy tests work and are they accurate?

On no, don't tell me...! If you're going to be sexually active you must take contraception more seriously. In the end it's down to you! When a woman becomes pregnant, initially tiny amounts of a special hormone called Human Chorionic Gonadotrophin (HCG) are released into her body to prepare the womb lining for the embryo to grow. Some of the HCG is naturally released into the urine. Biochemists have managed to create sensitive monoclonal antibodies which can detect the

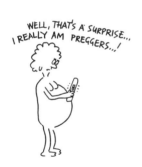

presence of this hormone from the first day of a missed period.

Pregnancy predictors all work in roughly the same way. They consist of a plastic pen-like device which is held into the morning's first urine stream. A dot or line appears in a small window should a pregnancy be recorded.

Predictors are relatively cheap to buy from any chemist and are very reliable. The makers claim 98-99 percent accuracy. Alcohol will not affect the reading, nor will medicines except special fertility drugs and some extremely rare medical conditions.

23. What and where is the G spot?

The G spot or Graefenburg spot, is a bit of a myth - it's not really a spot, more of an erogenous zone. It's the front of a woman's vagina behind the vaginal lips and clitoris. The walls of the vagina tend to be highly sensitive especially when aroused, that is when hormones and noradrenaline (Nature's own aphrodisiac) start to pump around the body.

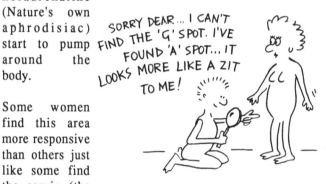

SORRY DEAR... I CAN'T FIND THE 'G' SPOT. I'VE FOUND 'A' SPOT... IT LOOKS MORE LIKE A ZIT TO ME!

Some women find this area more responsive than others just like some find the cervix (the neck of the womb) extremely sensitive - others don't think about it too much. They just get stuck in!

Did you know: There is a rare form of 'thrush' which can reside in the small intestine and grow little tentacles which burrow into the inner lining of the intestine.

Did you know: To make love in a car on a public right of way is indecent behaviour. It's OK if parked on private land and you're out of sight.

---

24. What's the cause of inverted nipples?

Many a young man has fumbled his way inside his girlfriend's blouse only to find her nipples are flat or inverted. What's wrong, he thinks, as he passionately tries to excite her...!

It's a very distressing situation for the young woman. She thinks something is wrong with her and that she's alone with this abnormality. In fact, flat or inverted nipples occur in about 10 percent of the female population... which represents something over two million women in the UK.

It's a very unfortunate condition which is largely heredity and permanent. According to a company in Suffolk called AVENT, which specialises in treatment of this condition, not a lot of research has been carried out on the subject.

Sudden nipple inversion (or nipples which do not 'stick out') can occur after surgery, an injury, from excessive weight or infection - these must be evaluated by a physician.

Nipples do come in different shapes and sizes - all of which are normal. Some are pendulous, some point in different directions - one could point up, the other down - some are even called 'mulberry nipples' which resemble small mulberries (similar to raspberries). They are all quite normal and as different as people's faces.

25. Do women release 'fluid', like men, when they have an orgasm?

Answers to this question have been kicking around for ages and out of all of the studies which have ben carried out, it's difficult to come to any positive conclusions.

When confronted with sexual experiences, both men and women tend to lie - especially when filling in questionnaires. They also tend to lie when being interviewed because they're naturally embarrassed. In a recent report, the British population will take part in virtually any survey on any subject but when it comes to sex, forget it. However, some scientists claim that with some women, a slight fluid release does occur on orgasm but evidence is a little weak. A small percentage have claimed an ejaculation - like experience from small glands at the vaginal opening but this might be tiny drops of urine being released as the pelvic area goes into a spasm. No one really knows the answer and as you can imagine, tests on climaxing women are few and far between.

Did you know: The term 'screwing' probably comes from the device used by farmers to artificially inseminate livestock. It is literally screwed into the animal's vagina to make the job easier.

Did you know: In a recent survey, 85 percent of adolescent girls said that they wanted to be thinner. 45 percent of boys said likewise.

26. I've heard of chastity belts for women, but is there a male equivalent?

The chastity belt, which was worn by women has been documented throughout history and worn until relatively recently.

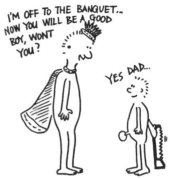

The belt which has a small padlock simply prevented women from having sexual intercourse. It was a drastic form of contraception but also prevented the spread of VD - especially syphilis (the pox), which was a major killer throughout Europe. The equivalent for males was infibulation which was achieved by putting a ring through the foreskin. Erection was extremely painful and intercourse, impossible. The words 'shall I give you a ring, sometime?' definitely had a different meaning in days gone by.

Did you know: The early Mexicans used extracts from the wild yam vine as a contraceptive. Modern commercial versions of the 'pill' were derived from this source by an American pharmaceutical company.

Did you know: Along the Pan American Highway in Alaska, there is a sign warning menstruating women and those wearing perfume to stay in their vehicles for fear of bear attacks.

27. I am taking anabolic steroids for a woman's body building competition. Will my sex life be affected?

All drugs have side effects on the human body. We've all seen photos of muscular, women body-builders which look more like men than men - and unfortunately, you stand a high risk in becoming more masculine by taking steroids. Firstly, there's the deeper voice, followed by acne and possible baldness - and irregular periods. But, on the plus side, you'll notice a larger clitoris and an increase in your sex drive! The amount of increase is obviously difficult to tell.

Many women will not mention any difference in their sex lives because of emotional, social, cultural and other taboos. All I can say is, be sensible. If you start developing a penis, you know you've been overdoing things.

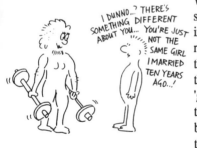

I DUNNO...? THERE'S SOMETHING DIFFERENT ABOUT YOU... YOU'RE JUST NOT THE SAME GIRL I MARRIED TEN YEARS AGO...!

When a man takes anabolic steroids, his sex drive will initially start to increase. This is not due to the drugs, it's simply that they feel more in control of their bodies. Anyone who looks 'good', feels good, especially if they had a flabby weak body before working out. However, the long term effects for both men and women can be very serious indeed: liver and kidney failure, diabetes, jaundice, osteoporosis and heart failure - a costly price to pay for a manly body and increased sex drive!

28. Do all women have a similar clitoris?

It's surprising what some women regard as normal. When it comes to comparison charts, sex organs and associated sundry items are not strongly featured. Each woman's clitoris is different in size and appearance and each one has no other role apart from providing stimulation and pleasure. Occasionally, a small or undeveloped clitoris can contribute to a lack of orgasm and the application of a male hormone cream may increase sexual response. Testosterone cream, if applied for some weeks, can increase the size and nerve/blood supply which can heighten s e n s i t i v i t y . Testosterone cream is not available in Britain but pharmacists can make you one up.

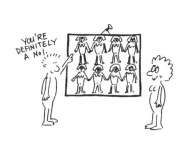

Of course there are other factors which affect clitoral performance. Psychological hang-ups such as being inhibited to 'let go', being scared and unwary and the fear of pregnancy - whether precautions are taken or not, all play a part.
Very, very few early sexual relationships end in orgasm for the woman: there is a learning process to achieving an orgasm which few young women realise!

29. My partner has been told he has 'thrush'. Can he pass it on to me?

If he starts calling his old dick 'tweety pie' and giving it bird seed, he's definitely got a bad case of thrush. It'll be bright red and very unfriendly. In men, thrush usually occurs as an irritating rash on the end of the penis or the whole of the genital area. It's sometimes called monilia and is a harmless yeast fungus that is present on all humans all of the time, but is usually controlled by our own immune systems.

Sometimes, such as when a person is taking antibiotics, the small organism mutates (candida albicans) and is not killed off and multiplies causing red hot itching. It can be passed on by sexual contact and can ping-pong between couples.

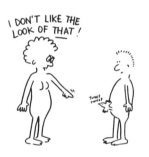

Tight jeans and nylon underpants should definitely be avoided. In women, thrush appears as a white, curd like vaginal discharge with the same red-hot itching. Needless to say, sexual intercourse becomes very painful indeed... it's a brave man who would even think of attempting such a thing with an affected partner!

So, can your partner pass it on to you? Yes he can. He's unlikely to want sex with a red hot and itchy penis (but you never know).

30. My man seems to have trouble in ejaculating... the whole business seems to go forever! What can I do to speed him up?

Some women would really envy you... after all, the average man ejacualates in far less than two minutes. It's only in films that the hero is a sexual athlete and can keep going for two hours!

Retarded ejaculation is uncommon and usually associated with the older man. The older a man gets, the less virile he is. He may take anything from half an hour to 24 hours before being able to manage a second ejaculation - even though he has an erection. A bit disconcerting to say the least!

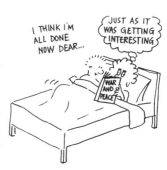

Your man may be tired or under stress; he may be taking medication which supresses the ejaculatory mechanism. He may be taking 'social' drugs such as marijuana or drinking too much alcohol. He could be influenced by a combination of any of these factors. Usually, delayed ejaculation is a temporary occurance. If it happens each time you make love, then disease to the prostate gland and nerves to the tiny ejaculatory muscles may be the cause.

31. Why do women have so many periods?

Periods are Nature's way of giving women a rest from the amorous pursuits of their menfolk. For most men, periods are a definite turn off, but not always...

Girls from about 12 - 50 years old have a period each month. They look worse than they feel - or is it - they feel worse that they look? Which ever way - a period is a bloody inconvenience!

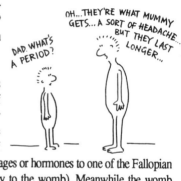

Every woman, from birth, has a fixed number of thousands of tiny eggs lodged in each of her two ovaries. Each month, the pituitary gland at the base of the brain, sends chemical messages or hormones to one of the Fallopian tubes (which connect the ovary to the womb). Meanwhile the womb lining thickens, hoping that a fertilised egg will attach itself to it. Every month it lives in hope. If the egg is not fertilised by a sperm, the egg, the lining of the womb and blood are simply not wanted and are jetisoned out through the vagina in a rather unceremonious way.

The amount of blood and tissue may look deceiving but in fact it's only about an eggcup full occurring over three or four days. All women experience 'different' periods: the duration, the amount of flow, the discomfort and lack of self-esteem, all vary. There's not much a woman can do to prevent herself from having a period. They're just part of being a woman.

32. I know a dog can smell a bitch on heat. Can men smell a woman who's having a period?

A man would have to get pretty close to smell a woman with a period. If he's allowed to get that close, he'll probably know her well enough to know her monthly cycle. Otherwise a sharp whack around the face would soon direct his sniffing elsewhere.

Menstrual blood does have a slight odour but so do all our body fluids. Personal hygiene is of great importance because bacteria soon set in and make a meal of any excretions. It's important to bathe or shower regularly and tampons should be changed at least every four hours, that way you can be completely confident.

Dogs can smell a bitch on heat because they're supposed to! Chemicals are released, automatically, to excite any passing dog to mate. It's the only time when animals have sexual intercourse... of course, we humans are far 'luckier' and can enjoy sexual encounters whenever we choose. Well virtually...

Did you know: A rare and bizarre side effect of the anti-depressant Anafranil was reported in three patients. They claimed that every time they yawned they achieved an orgasm. They didn't state whether they were male or female. Anafranil is available only on prescription.

Did you know: Men ejaculate between three to seven times during orgasm at a rate of 1.25 times per second.

---

33. Do men have changes in their hormone levels each month like women?

Some men have changes in their hormone levels every night! Research has shown that men <u>do</u> have a hormonal cycle. It isn't so acute as for women and varies from between 8-30 days depending upon the individual. Why testosterone (the main sex hormones) and other hormones in the blood vary, scientists just don't know and research is being carried out on cyclic variations in male hormones. One thing scientists do know : the same fluctuating levels of hormones affect men differently. Some feel sexier, some more aggressive, some more depressed. Why this is so, is still a mystery.

So next time your boss gets all moody and shouts at you, just spread the fact that his biorhythms are playing him up and he's not feeling himself. (Perhaps he'd be able to relax a little if he did feel himself!).

A brand new form of contraception has been offered for sale in Los Angeles. It's even more effective than the pill - claim the manufacturers. It's called 'Baby Think It Over' and is a life like replica of a 3.6 kg human baby which emits an earpiercing scream at random intervals. Inserting a key in the baby's back and nursing it for 30 minutes is the only way to stop the screaming. After being given the 'baby' for a week, hundreds of schoolgirls have vowed never to have children! America!

Did you know: One in three British pregnancies is unplanned.

34. Why are men's balls all crinkly?

Actually, their balls aren't all crinkly - they're quite firm and roundish. It's the scrotum that holds them that has that odd texture. It's all 'crinkly' because sperm manufacture requires a slightly lower temperature than the rest of the body. The skin needs to be able to shrink and expand quickly in order to keep an optimum temperature of about 3-4 degrees F below body temperature.

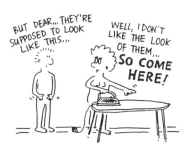

Consequently, it's made from loose skin - the thinner it is, the more flexible it is. Also, the loose skin hanging away from the body enables as much air as possible to circulate around the testicles to try to keep them cooler. Why this temperature is critical is anyone's guess (I expect someone out there knows!).

The scrotum has to be loose and hanging to allow as much blood as possible to flow to the fine network of tubes inside each testis without being too constricted. Unfortunately, there is a hitch: the testes can become twisted and cut off the blood supply! It usually happens in young men between 13-16 years old; presumably because they are more physically active. An emergency operation is necessary to prevent irreversible damage.

35. Do men have erogenous zones like women?

Of course they do, and like most women, men only respond when they're with someone who turns them on: they are generally less selective though. Men like to be kissed, have their ears, neck, inner thighs and arms gently stroked and kissed.

They like their backs and shoulders rubbed, their spines vigorously massaged and their balls gently handled. Of course one erogenous zone sticks out a mile: men like to have the top of their penis sucked or kissed and the shaft of the penis gently stroked (well, that's a new one on me!).

Did you know: In studies of computer dating questionaires, women evaluate potential partners far more closely than men. Attributes such as status, religious views, intelligence and background play a large part in selection. Physical attractiveness did not seem to matter. With men, attractiveness, youth and a good figure were top of the list.

Did you know: The word 'bonk' was originally used in the First World War. It means to shell or continually hit - in a military sense. The media today presumably think it sounds raunchy enough to give it a new meaning.

Did you know: Approximately 19,000,000,000 contraceptive pills are swallowed around the world every year.

36. I heard that a woman can't get pregnant by having sexual intercourse while standing up. Is this true?

Are you kidding me? There's no stopping those sperm once they get moving. They're like greyhounds on steroids which defy the laws of gravity. With well over 200 million of them released at once, there's always one that can find his way in the dark without a map!

Of course most of his mates will fall by the wayside - or in your case, fall onto the floor. However a large

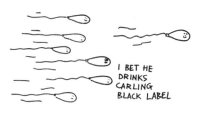

I BET HE DRINKS CARLING BLACK LABEL

group will end up in the cervical mucus, trapped and suspended. There will always be a few who struggle free and find their way pass the womb to the Fallopian tubes ready to fertilise a waiting egg. They even have minute little motors behind their heads to give them extra energy and a long whip-like tail. They're lethal. In fact, in tests, sperm have been recorded in the Fallopian tubes half an hour after intercourse. OK it's only a distance of about 15 cms (6 ins) but that's like an Olympic athlete running two marathons at 60 miles an hour. Think about it...

Don't listen to any more rumours about not getting pregnant - they're probably not true. Protect yourself or your partner and take some form of contraception.

37. Is it true that a man can get cancer of the penis?

Cancer is not a very nice word. There are over 200 types of cancer which can affect the human body in one form or another. And yes, a man's dingle dangle can offer very little resistance. Thankfully, cancer of the penis or penile cancer is rare - comprising less than three percent of all cancers.

Initially the cancer starts as a painless wart or nasty ulcer on the tip of the penis and gradually develops along the shaft in a series of painful lesions. Surgery is definitely called for and I won't let you know what surgeons have to do - but I think you can guess! It can bring tears to your eyes just thinking about it. Still, it is pretty uncommon and usually only affects those men who have been sleeping rough for a long time. Tramps are likely candidates and the cancer seems to be brought on by a virus - but no one really knows for sure.

In Uganda, penile cancer is the most common cause of cancer in men. If you're thinking of chucking everything in and living a life on the road in sunny Uganda - be warned.

Did you know: The word vagina is derived from the latin word 'halter' - somewhere a Roman soldier stuck his sword.

Did you know: It's estimated that at every second 19,000 men are ejaculating somewhere around the world: this excludes the D.I.Y. jobs!

Did you know: A woman who is taking fertility drugs stands a 12 - 15 per cent chance of having twins, triplets or multiple births.

---

38. Why do some women get all depressed after having a baby?

Some women get depressed because they realise they should have taken some contraceptive precautions months ago. And now look... heavy breathing one minute... a baby the next! Post natal depression occurs in about 5-10 percent of women - some of these might require hospitalisation if the symptoms are really severe.

Even after a few months of giving birth, the new mother may find herself tired, irritable, useless, lacking any self motivation, guilty, sexless and pitifully depressed. What's more, she may know she's like this but can't seem to understand why.

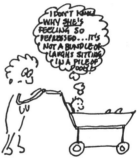

Well, we're back to hormones again! The low levels of oestrogen and progesterone can cause some of these problems and the feelings of isolation may aggravate the whole situation. Imagine the exhausting task of looking after a new-born baby around the clock... the unreasonable attitude of a partner - or the lack of any supportive partner... the possible financial uncertainties of bringing up the baby... the restrictions of being confined to the house or flat and on top of that, everyone expects you to feel great!

39. My wife's vagina is just too big - my penis seems to get lost in it. What can I do to help her?

Your dick's too limp! The problem of a sagging vagina is common in some women - especially after bearing several children. The vagina becomes overstretched and simply loses its youthful grip. Not only does this cause some sexual impairment for the man, it also causes reduced satisfaction for the woman.

The man complains that his penis doesn't seem to touch the sides because his partner's vaginal muscles are too weak to grasp the penis shaft firmly. Consequently, the woman becomes frustrated that her clitoris doesn't get fully aroused on intercourse. She can try sitting astride you or closing her legs during love making: this will temporarily overcome the problem but the real 'cure' is to tighten up the pelvic floor muscle which runs from the back passage to the front passage! There are various toning up exercises that can be done by contracting and releasing this large pubococcygeus muscle. It's up to her to perform this at least 200 times a day by squeezing and releasing her vaginal lips!

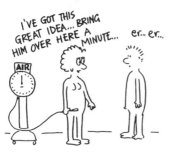

A high-fibre diet can also reduce constipation which in itself tends to push down on this muscle. A tighter muscle won't happen overnight and might take several months - repeated exercises are paramount.

40. Do men desire more sexual variety than women?

Men do tend to have a 'never let a chance go by' attitude when it comes to mating. Their ability to have rapid erections means that should the opportunity arise, they are able to pass their their genes on to as many women as possible. It's a primary function of being a male. So yes, men will always desire more novelty - or perhaps a better word would be 'variety'.

Of course, in modern civilised societies, restraints are put on our behaviour but the innate mating instincts are still there. Erotic pictures can act as a substitute, enabling the man to fantasise copulation with the woman in the picture. Almost all pornography is designed and bought by men, in order to capitalise on this sexual need.

Women, on the other hand are also aroused by erotic, rather than pornographic pictures. They are naturally more selective when choosing a mate. Let's face it, they have to be: there has always been a lot of dross around and the woman has to be sure that she's going to be cared for whilst being heavily pregnant. So, a woman's sexual fantasies mean that stories which show couples caring, loving and caressing are far more arousing. It's this natural instinct which means romance novels are written mainly by women, for women. They just fulfil a basic need.

When you see a man leering over a girlie magazine, just remember it's all to do with his stoneage mentality. When you next see a woman smiling while reading a slushy romance nove, remember-she's really broody and needs a 'real' man to look after her!

41. Why do some women go off sex?

Imagine, having the same old meal at the same restaurant day after day. After a while, your tastebuds don't get turned on. In some ways, sex can be just the same. Some women would find staying up late to see the test card on TV more stimulating!

Men are usually obsessed with an erect penis but routine and fatigue can get the better of every couple as the years pass by.

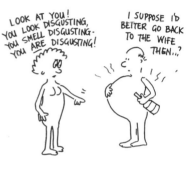

LOOK AT YOU! YOU LOOK DISGUSTING, YOU SMELL DISGUSTING. YOU ARE DISGUSTING!

I SUPPOSE I'D BETTER GO BACK TO THE WIFE THEN...?

The man may have a certain amount of stress inflicted upon him - simply to cope with the financial demands of his teenage family. He comes home late, only to find his partner barely able to function with the day to day running of the home and the children's needs. Then there's the headaches, the periods, the menopause and the in-laws to contend with...

Just when the woman needs a few words of love and affection before sleeping, the man wants to get it all over and done with before he falls asleep on the job! Also, in relationships there can be mixed feelings of anger and resentment towards one's partner. Sometimes these feelings may be derived from long-standing and deep conflicts that have been exggerated out of all proportion over the years.

Consequently, the woman can deny any sexual favours to her man as a cruel 'punishment'. More often than not, the man may not even know that he's done or said anything wrong. It's all very distressing. Life is so short and in the end, happiness is all we have. But the whole situation just festers until both partners just accept things without talking the problem over. They imagine that all couples feel the same! And then there's the woman who doesn't find her partner attractive any longer. Maybe she was coerced into marriage or the relationship at an early age. Again, sexual desire can be used as punishment towards the man through feelings of guilt on her behalf.

Sexual desire does come and go over the years as family responsibilities increase. The man may be influenced by attractive, younger women at the office and he can easily draw comparisons which are totally unfair. His partner can be made to feel sexless and physically way past her sell by date. Depression can set in and a depressed woman is hardly a bundle of laughs - let alone a sexual tornado!

Some men (and women) develop unsavoury and disgusting personal habits over the years which can play havoc with anyone's sex life. Obesity is another turn off especially when stale sweat is in the air. Some men might expect too much and judge the total worth of their lives on their sexual prowess and virility. Their partners might not be able to see this and only want the occasional sensual words of excitement rather than a full frontal attack.

So, really there are many reasons why men and women 'go off sex'. Some may be far more complex than the reasons I've mentioned and some may deteriorate rapidly or painfully slowly.

42. My wife keeps accusing me of having erotic dreams (with someone else in mind) because I still have wet dreams. What can I do to tell her she's wrong?

Yes, she may also think she's not satisfying you enough. More frequent sexual intercourse may reduce emissions. You must tell her (or show her this book) that wet dreams are involuntary spasms that occur at any age (see Q8). Naturally she may feel inadequate and accuse you of erotic dreaming because she dosen't want to reveal her true thoughts. There's no way of stopping wet dreams and the ejaculations may not be even sexually motivated at all.

The average man produces between 70 - 80 million sperm a day. Seminal fluid is also being produced to keep them all healthy: they can't all be absorbed so readily back into the body and sometimes an overload occurs. Unfortunately for your wife, it's all over the bedsheets.

Perhaps she's really annoyed at the fact she has to keep washing them!

Did You Know: Some moths can smell a female moth flying up to seven miles (12km) away.

Did you know: A baby is born somewhere in the world every quarter of a second and every year almost 100 million more people are born than die.

Did you know: 2.5 percent of girls never tell their mothers of their first period.

43. My man is sex mad. Is there anything which I can give him to slow him down a bit?

I know, I know, you can take it but it's his health you are worried about. And no, he's definitely not as young or as thin as he used to be! Think of his heart... Having said that, you could fatten him up a lot more. Men who are too fat have high levels of the female hormone - oestradiol, in their bodies, which suppresses sexual desire, performance and fertility.

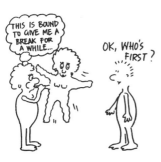

But then, this hormone can lead to heart and blood vessel disease. There are drugs that do reduce sexual desire : these are given to sex offenders but don't always work. Obviously they're not freely available. Other drugs which control anxiety, hay fever, ulcers, bladder infections, malaria and high blood pressure also reduce sexual libido. I wouldn't recommend you to hand any of these out as there are always side-effects.

There is bromine - which was used in the Second World War to keep soldiers minds on fighting the enemy and not fighting their sexual desires. How you obtain it, I just don't know. There are natural tranquillisers available which might make him feel less tense, foods containing magnesium, vitamin B1, vitamin B6 and B3, vitamin C, for instance. But then, these might make him too relaxed and ready for 'anything'!

44. My man keeps on complaining about having a pain on erection. What's wrong with him?

I remember hearing of a young man who, whilst out late with his mates, desperately wanted to relieve himself. Their car stopped. He leapt out and almost immediately there was a horrific scream. He accidentally placed his penis on an electrified fence. Talk about a shock... his dick hasn't been the same since!

But your man's erection has nothing to do with electric fences - unless he's the same man as in the story! (By the way, the story is true. How could I forget it?). I know it's embarrassing but he should really go and visit his physician. He'll probably tell him he's got

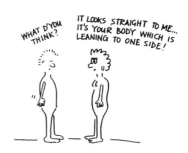

WHAT D'YOU THINK?

IT LOOKS STRAIGHT TO ME... IT'S YOUR BODY WHICH IS LEANING TO ONE SIDE!

Peyronie's disease. It happens in middle-aged or older men and the penis tends to bend rather acutely to one side when erect. It's impossible to straighten and makes intercourse a non-event. No one really knows what causes it, but it's the build up of tissue on one side of the penis shaft. One side gets a blood supply-and consequently gets rigid, but the other side becomes blocked. It's very painful and apparently can be brought on by injury during vigorous sexual activity!

45. Why do men have two testicles and not just one big one?

Yes? And why not have half a dozen? They could hang down like a bunch of grapes - all purple and crinkly in the noon day sun! Nature endowed human beings with virtually two of everything. I suppose we could have done with two hearts and in some cases a back-up brain may be useful... and testicles are just the same. Injury to one testicle would enable the other to work successfully so primitive man would still remain fertile. Diseases such as epidynitis can happen to any man-especially older men, and testicular cysts can affect one testicle at any time, again as a result of injury or infection. In the case of torsion of the testis, the spermatic cord becomes twisted, for no apparent reason, but the other testis can still function properly.

Reproduction has always been high on the list of Nature's priorities. The man is writhing around in agony but Nature didn't care - she just wanted sperm production no matter what. Let's face it, a real man wouldn't have even batted an eyelid should one testicle be half-severed by a sabre tooth tiger or speared by a sharp thorn... There must be a design flaw here: I reckon we should have been pollinated by bees!

Did you know: In 1833 the average age for a girl to have her first period was 17. Today, it's 12. Nutrition and body weight have played a big part in bringing about this change.

Did you know: 30% of couples in Britain now co-habitat rather than marry.

---

46. Are those new female condoms any good?

What d'you mean? any good? They're certainly good at stopping pregnancies and preventing HIV and STD infections. They don't come in flavours and they're like condoms except instead of covering the penis they line the vagina. They're made from super-strong polyurethane and inserted rather like a tampon.

There's a margin all around which covers the vaginal entrance.

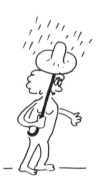
However they do tend to be a bit noisy because they rustle a bit. Some women complain of feeling uncomfortable whilst others have difficulty inserting them properly. But the failure rate if used proficiently is as low as the male condom. They are incredibly fine and so both men and women are assured of a great deal of sensitivity. If you fancy rustling up something a little different for your sex life, why not buy some? I'm sure you can find other uses for them if you change your mind!

Did you know: Two of the UK's major airlines claim there is no such thing as the Mile High Club. If you know differently, I'd like to know!.

Did you know: In Kansas and Massachusetts, USA, girls can marry at the age of twelve, with parental consent.

Did you know: In 1994, in the UK, 9000 girls under the age of 16 had babies.

47. Where did AIDS come from?

We've all heard about HIV and AIDS: the disease and its social implications have been widely publicised. The HIV (Human Immunodeficiency Virus) which can lead to AIDS has probably been around for a long time. Its source was probably in remote rural populations of Central Africa where it is still known as Slim Disease because of the wasting effects it has on the human body.

People don't die directly from AIDS but from the resulting debilitating diseases such as pneumonia, rare cancers, brain damage and other infections. A virus very similar to the HIV virus was first discovered in the African green monkey but it didn't seem to have any ill effects. However, in macaque monkeys, it caused a similar effect to AIDS. How the virus was passed on to humans is open to speculation. It could have been through being bitten, scratched, eating the meat, 'unnatural' sexual practices or in witchcraft rites.

Certainly there were many cases of AIDS in Zaire, Uganda and Kenya and from here it probably spread to other parts of Africa and then to the Caribbean, namely Haiti.

Homosexual men are very mobile and consequently AIDS established itself into the large America gay community. Intravenous drug abusers in New York then contracted the virus and soon donors blood became contaminated. World-wide infection spread rapidly and now no country is AIDS free.

48. Why does the ability to climax vary so much from woman to woman?

It varies so much because they are women. Orgasm in women varies between individuals and sexual arousal is linked with changes in the menstrual cycles, age and the type of relationship a woman is in. Also hormonal changes in the menopause, pregnancy and after childbirth have a major effect on behaviour and sexual desire.

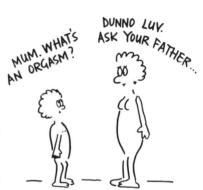

However, the physiological responses in women are the same. Initially blood flows to the clitoris and surrounding area making the vagina secrete a fluid type mucus from the vaginal walls. In this excitement stage the pelvic blood supply continues and the vaginal lips become congested with blood. The clitoris enlarges and the vaginal lips move outwards and upwards to reveal the vaginal opening. At this stage, the woman's heart beat increases. This excitement stage varies and older women find vaginal lubrication still occurs but it just takes longer. Most women find their breasts and nipples enlarge and their womb swells and is lifted upwards. All this takes about 30 seconds and can vary depending upon their general mental and physical health.

This excitement stage is followed by a plateau stage when the inner deeper part of the vagina begins to enlarge upwards. The lower vagina becomes tighter so enabling a firmer grip of the penis and the clitoris starts to shrink. The inner lips or labia minora change from a lightish pink through to a deep burgundy red as more blood flows to the pelvic region. The clitoris becomes extremely sensitive round about now and the whole body feels stimulated with a further increase in pulse rate, blood pressure and dilation of the pupils. Again, this level of excitement varies, it can peak and trough and depends on further factors such as sexual experience and knowing what to expect! The orgasmic or myotonic stage definitely varies from woman to woman. There is an increase in muscle tension-especially in the pelvic region and there is a series of rapid contractions in the lower one third of the vagina. Sometimes there are involuntary muscle spasms in other parts of the body creating wave-like sensations that we call an orgasm! The average orgasm lasts from 10-15 seconds but again this can vary and a woman may experience further orgasms if they're lucky!

Many women feel that an orgasm is not really necessary on sexual intercourse. They still feel they have happy sex lives and enjoy making their partner feel happy and relaxed. Surveys of married women show that 22-74 percent usually experience orgasm during intercourse, 30-45 percent experience it occasionally and 5-22 percent never experience it. Rarely do both partners experience relief at the same time.

49. What's a prostate gland and why don't women have them?

Women have enough reproductive bits and pieces inside them! They all have their fair share of going wrong at times and so Nature introduced the prostate gland for men, to redress the balance.

The prostate is a walnut sized gland which sits just below the bladder. It's responsible for producing most of the semen in which sperm are able to swim and be nourished on their somewhat hostile journey. In older men, the prostate can 'play up' and cause havoc with a normal sex life. It can become inflamed, become enlarged or even cancerous. The prostate gland pushes down directly onto the tube which leads from the bladder to the penis and any problems with the prostate automatically affect urinating.

Did you know: In a list of teenage priorities, a recent study of 1000 New York young adults revealed that having sexual intercourse was rated at No 13 for girls and No 8 for boys. Finding a job was top of the list for both boys and girls.

Did you know: It's estimated that at any one moment, six million couples are copulating somewhere around the world.

Did you know: The maximum number of recorded births for one woman is 69. A Russian woman, Feodor Vassilet (1708 - 1782) had several sets of triplets and quadruplets, only two didn't live to adulthood.

50. Do infertile men make poor lovers?

Well, it all depends what you call a poor lover - or more to the point, what you call a good lover.

An infertile man is physically no different from any other man. He still produces the same amount of semen, has erections in just the same way and ejaculates like other men. It's just that the sperm in his semen are not up to standard or there are simply not enough. In many societies, fertility is compared with virility: the two are completely different but myths die hard. The speed of erection and size of a willie can be very misleading when it comes to fertility.

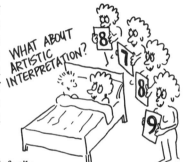

When a man first learns of being infertile, yes, he can naturally be anxious to the point of not wanting sex. If he wants to father children, the pressures and stress levels, coupled with lack of self-esteem and failure, are very traumatic.

External attitudes from friends, parents, in-laws and sometimes his partner can lead to an uncontrollable sense of guilt. No man can expect to be a superstud under such mental torment. And, the problem is just the same for women, in fact harder. Every month she is reminded of her womanly instinct to reproduce. Sexual intercourse can seem pointless and her infertility problems can lead to a very negative attitude towards sex.

51. My husband sometimes gets an erection at odd times for no apparent reason. Why is this?

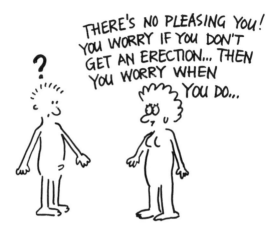

THERE'S NO PLEASING YOU! YOU WORRY IF YOU DON'T GET AN ERECTION... THEN YOU WORRY WHEN YOU DO...

As I said before, happiness is what you think... in this case, unhappiness is what you don't think! Painful and prolonged erection without sexual arousal is called priapism. It can be brought on by taking certain medicines, by spinal cord injuries or sickle cell disease.

He must visit his doctor urgently. Treatment may involve withdrawal of blood from the penis with a syringe! If he leaves the condition untreated, he could end up impotent. In fact, any incidence of pain in the penis or blood in the semen should be referred to a doctor immediately.

52. What do they mean by female circumcision?

The answer to this question will definitely put you off your dinner! Female circumsion involves removing the clitoris of a young woman who has not yet started her periods.

This is practiced in many parts of the world as an initiation rite to welcome a girl into womanhood. It is usually performed by other women of a tribe or family, by removing the clitoris with a sharp knife or stick! An anaesthetic is not used and infection often occurs.

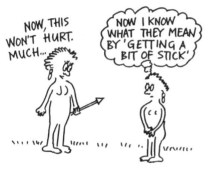

West African countries regard female circumcision as a way of reducing the sex-drive in women. Also, by curbing sexual pleasure, it's thought that a woman will be less inclined to seek extra-marital relationships. Well, the clitoris does play a big part in sexual satisfaction but the sex drive is determined by hormones being released by the pituitary gland. The whole practice is trying to be discouraged by international agencies because of the risk of blood contamination and the AIDS epidemic.

53. I want to be a virgin when I marry so how do I know if my hymen is still intact?

It you're prodding and probing around your nether regions looking for the elusive hymen you could be virgin on an impossible task. Virginity is determined by sexual intercourse not by whether your hymen is still intact. Obviously the two can be related and in some countries, a marriage is only considered to be consummated if a few drops of blood are present on the wedding sheets the following morning. This is a myth and in reality, a few drops of animal blood often make do. You see, not all virgins have an intact hymen.

These days, the hymen can rupture and be non-existent before puberty. Young girls can be very active and cycling, tree climbing, using tampons, ice skating, horse riding and other activities can easily tear the hymen without the girl even knowing. She might be using tampons to soak up menstrual blood and a few drops of extra blood from the broken hymen will not even be detected. Masturbation with an object can also cause a hymen to rupture. After all, the hymen is just a soft membrane around the vaginal opening. Sometimes it covers the whole opening to the vagina but in some girls, only small ragged remains can be seen. In other words, the hymen varies from person to person... some can even be multiple or crescent shaped. It all depends.

No one really knows what the hymen is supposed to do: it's of no medical significance and in many ways can only restrict menstrual blood early on in a woman's life.

But still old rumours exist. Some girls believe that the first time wicked willie says hello, intercourse will be quite painful, but normally in all virgins, only part of the hymen, if none at all will remain. Penetration shouldn't be painful at all. However, sometimes an imperforate hymen can cause a problem. The penis is simply unable to make any headway. The hymen is just too elastic and no amount of thrusting and throbbing will make any difference! This is a very rare situation and can be easily remedied by a doctor, a few reassuring words and a large machete!

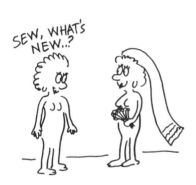

Some societies are so obsessed with pre-marital purity that the ragged remains of a woman's hymen can be re-stitched in order to make her marriageable. A stitch in time can save a lot of unnecessary embarrassment later!

Did you know: 4 percent of couples in Britain claim to make love once a day.

Did you know: In Britain it's illegal to be tattooed on the breasts, thighs - or anywhere else on the body until the age of 18. (Tattooing of Minors Act, 1969).

54. I heard that some women don't have periods. Is this true?

Yes it is true: they're called old! No, that's unfair. Women who are past the menopause cease to have any periods at all unless they're on HRT treatment. Lack of any periods - even from puberty is called amenorrhoea. Some women are born without a womb which makes having a period impossible. Sometimes periods stop for many different reasons and ten percent of women experience episodes of amenorrhoea at some time during their reproductive life.

In most instances, hormones are to blame. (They're a cause of a lot of things as we're finding out!). The pituitary gland stops sending signals for an egg to be released. No egg, no period. Usually this is because of severe weight loss (anorexia), excessive exercise, becoming overweight or sudden trauma or stress, but blockages in the womb or vaginal cysts may also be the cause.

There are other factors such as tumours or some women fail to have periods once they come off the contraceptive pill.Of course periods do become less and less and finally stop.

Many women think if their periods aren't regular then waste products or poisons build up in the body. This is quite untrue and their health won't be affected at all. It's always best to get checked over if this ever occurs though.

55. How often do condoms split during making love?

Some couples have very hectic sex lives that can be quite demanding on a super-thin area of latex rubber: teeth, whip marks and nails can always be damaging and some rectums are tighter than others! Usually the condom is extremely safe - providing it is removed carefully from the wrapper and used properly. Under 'normal' circumstances, the condom is 98 percent effective. It will not split at all: stringent manufacturing methods ensure this. Some men complain that sensitivity becomes impaired: 'It's like wearing a Wellington Boot,' they claim. This is ridiculous, but with some men no amount of argument will change their beliefs.

Other men complain they are too baggy!... but there are condoms on the market which are narrower. However, there is not an extra large condom on the market! It's important that the condom remains tight on the penis to prevent leakage after ejaculation. (That's where the 2 percent failure rate comes in). Semen can get all over the place when having intercourse: It's a damp nuisance which condoms help to prevent.

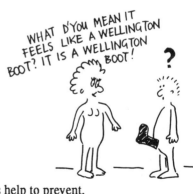

63
---

56. Why does my husband just turn over and go to sleep after our love making?

Some women wish their husbands would go to sleep as soon as their heads hit the pillow! Men can be many things in bed; arrogant, selfish and above all, ignorant, when it comes to sex! They think that they know how to please a woman, that they must always make the first move, that any talking before hand ruins the spontaneity, that it's not macho to express their feelings, that their partner always has multiple orgasms at exactly the same time as them and worst of all, many think that they know exactly

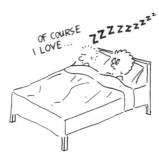

OF COURSE I LOVE... ZZZzzzzzᶻᶻ

what their partner is thinking - as if by some superhuman instinct! Put any or all of these beliefs together and you have a Neanderthal cocktail of sexual behaviour. The primary instinct to mate comes to the surface and once that's over... well it's over. It's time to rest until the opportunity arises again.

There is a short time (a refractory period) after ejaculating that a man is incapable of being sexually aroused. This might last from two to 30 minutes. As men become older this period intends to increase and they are in a natural state of relaxation. If a man is overweight, tired, stressed or a physical wreck, then his body tends to 'shut down' and sleep can occur rapidly. Sexual tension has been relieved and the brain also needs to rest.

Of course the same happens to a woman but she has a longer refractory period. Generally a woman takes longer to become aroused and longer to return to her natural state (approximately six minutes). So unfortunately a woman may wish to be gently caressed, talk and be close while her partner may not feel like doing anything but sleeping after intercourse. It's not really his 'fault' it's just a physiological difference that the man may not recognise.

Communication is the key. You cannot expect your husband to know what you're thinking - even after a life time of marriage. He may think he knows what you're thinking but this is not necessarily so, as we've just mentioned. Talk to him and tell him how you feel - it may prove to be a good investment.

Did you know: 23 percent of women in Britain are taking the contraceptive pill.

Did you know: Oysters change their sex twice throughout their lives. They are born female, change to male and then revert to being female - (No wonder they have psychiatric problems).

57. My boyfriend keeps pestering me to have sex with him. I am 16 and I know it has to happen some time. Should I wait or get it over and done with?

Many young men will say and do anything to get their own way. They want to prove they are 'real' men - all grown up - and to be able to boast about their sexual exploits. You are just a pawn in the game. Believe me, he only has his own interests at heart. OK, your fella isn't like that! Oh yeah? You just wait till he's with his mates... I can almost hear your name being mentioned... a real push over... a sex mad nympho... and worse!

Obviously that's not the way you'll see it but young men will always be young men! Just the fact that he's pestering you must make you realise what his true nature is like. If he were sincere and cared, he'd let you take your time until you thought the time was right.

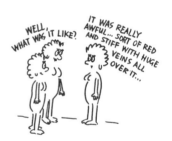

You will remember your first sexual intercourse for the rest of your life: don't let it be a pressurised, hasty act of regret.

Many young men and women feel that 'sex' is a thing to try and losing one's virginity is a step that has to be taken sometime. Friends harrass each other and often 14 and 15 year old girls are made to feel left out if they haven't had intercourse. It's definitely regarded as abnormal to be a virgin at 18! Relationships built on such flimsy ground are bound to collapse: remember you're in charge.

58. Are men more romantic than women?

Men do think of romance differently from women; their primary instinct is to mate. Many a young man will say and do virtually anything 'romantic' to get his wicked willie into action. His romantic inclinations are tied up with his sexual intentions. However, a woman's romantic inclinations are linked with emotional attachment and a need to be close - but not necessarily that close!

Women want to cuddle and caress, while men want to

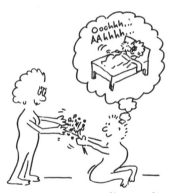

exceed this point and, well... I think you know what I'm getting at! In an American study however, students were asked to disagree or agree with:"True love is to be in love forever". Far more men agreed with this statement than women. But, of course romantic ideals do not necessarily translate into romantic behaviour! In Western society, we're fortunate in being able to express romantic feelings. We are at the extreme end of sexual intimate display and togetherness. So the word romance means many things to many people... men write most love songs; women read most romantic novels. Who is the more romantic? Both are equal: but in different ways.

59. What's the difference between PMS and PMT? Why do only some women suffer?

Many people think that PMS and PMT are the same thing: they're not. PMS is premenstrual syndrome and encompasses many emotional and physical symptoms which occur in the middle of the monthly cycle of a reproductive-aged woman. PMT is premenstrual tension which brings on anxiety, irritability and sometimes aggression around the time a woman is having her period.

PMS is surprisingly common and 70 percent of women report some kind of emotional and physical changes in the middle of their cycle after they've released an egg (ovulated). Two to five percent of women experience severely distressing premenstrual symptoms world-wide. PMS does not respect race, colour, intelligence or socio-economic status.

Women are physiologically different from men and are subjected to changes in the metabolism due to the effects of their hormone cycles. (Men produce male hormones in their testicles as a constant flow).

The symptoms of PMS can range from depression, loss of self-esteem, insomnia, feelings of guilt, sudden angry outbursts, lack of concentration and being moody. Painful breasts, fluid retention, weight gain, headaches, dizziness, a craving for sugary foods and the flaring up of skin problems, such as acne and herpes can all be associated with PMS. But other serious diseases can masquerade as PMS - for example thyroid, pituitary and adrenal gland disorders. So it's important for PMS sufferers to keep a menstrual chart which describes accurate symptoms. Symptoms which are constant can be isolated from PMS and treated accordingly. Some women with personality disorders or severe depression may attribute these symptoms to PMS and fail to seek correct treatment.

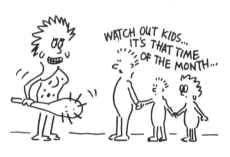

The symptoms of PMS are more obvious than the actual cause. Clinical research points to a subtle reduction in oestrogen and more importantly progesterone in the middle of a woman's cycle as the primary cause of PMS. These female hormones are necessary to stimulate the release of an egg and are controlled by the pituitary gland in the front part of the brain. Everything is interlinked and any imbalances in the fine tuning can play havoc in the rest of a woman's body.

60. Do middle-aged women have sex less often than younger women?

Despite everything that has been written or said about sex and the older woman, Dr Sandra Cabot, who founded the Australian Woman's Health Advisory Service, reports that a sexual interest remains eternal in the majority of women.

There is a reduced sex drive in the menopausal years because of a reduction in sex hormones. This can lead to the womb shrinking and the vagina losing its elasticity and lubrication. At this time sex can become unwelcome and painful.

LUBRICATION? HOW ABOUT THIS?

But there are treatments which can rectify this and even a vaginal oestrogen cream that can restore vaginal youthfulness!

During middle age (whenever that is!) and beyond, both men and women take longer to reach orgasm so love-making takes on a slower pace. It becomes warmer and more 'meaningful'...it dosen't really matter whether the woman reaches a climax. Sex becomes fun without all the emotional hang-ups that can create problems in younger couples.

61. Why can't they find a contraceptive pill for men. I mean, why should women be the responsible sex all the time?

You're right. Most forms of preventing pregnancy are left up to the woman. Men do have a choice: a vasectomy - which is a bit drastic or using condoms which some men refuse to use.

Scientists are trying to find a contraceptive pill for men which limits their sperm production. Tests have been carried out but proved to be successful in just over half of men. The side effects included a feeling of weakness and nausea. And research suggests that this method of contraception would be very unpopular with men. They tend to regard pregnancy - and avoiding pregnancy as a woman's issue!

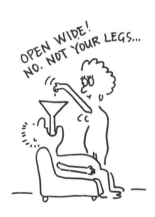

A well known woman's magazine recently asked its readers "Would you trust a man who said he took the pill?" A positive 'no' was the reply with suggestions that men were irresponsible and couldn't be trusted. There were some replies that said they would only trust a man if the pill turned the whites of his eyes green or pink! Women wanted a visual indication of a man's word.

62. What is Vatican Roulette?

Some religions around the world are very strict about contraception and they object to any form being used.

Although this situation is easing a lot, some couples have to become brilliant at curtailing their sexual impulses and leave lovemaking to about ten days each month. The rest of the time they 'improvise'!

Every month, all pre-menopausal women release a tiny egg from one of their two ovaries. Some women can feel a dull pain on one side of their body when this happens. It occurs about two weeks before her period starts and her body temperature increases about 1°c. A few days before this she is at her most fertile and can easily become pregnant. Apart from this rise in temperature, her cervical mucus, high up in the vagina, turns form being thin and watery to cloudy, thick and sticky. Sperm can live in this sticky mucus waiting for a chance to fertilise the egg in the Fallopian tube. It acts as a kind of reservoir because the egg can only live for a day and Nature wanted to

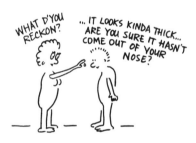

give women the best chance to conceive. After 24 hours the mucus becomes even thicker and the sperm can't move. This is now a safe time to have intercourse.

Changes in cervical mucus can be detected with the fingers. It takes a lot of practice because vaginal mucus and vaginal fluid (released on sexual arousal) all tend to dilute things. Recognising changes in mucus is a hit and miss affair and that's why it's called Vatican Roulette. The word Vatican is obviously connected with the Roman Catholic religion but this safe or rhythm form of contraception is not necessarily restricted to this religious faith.

Today, in the West, there is a urinary 'dip stick' which can easily detect when a woman is releasing an egg by hormonal changes which show up in her urine. Unfortunately though, women in many parts of the world can't afford to buy such luxuries - even if they were obtainable. For them Vatican Roulette and a bit (or a lot) of luck is all they rely on, not to become pregnant. A 20 percent failure rate is very common and until contraceptive barriers are lifted, the world population will continue to rise.

The oldest mother in Britain is a 59 year old: the oldest in the world is Rosa Della Corte, aged 62. She recently gave birth to a healthy son. (His first words were not 'Mummy' or 'Granny' but 'Why me?'!)

Did you know: There are about 150 million pregnant women in the world at any one time.

63. Is it true that some women are allergic to condoms?

Human beings can be allergic to a whole range of things. Allergic reactions can be brought on at any time usually by certain foodstuffs and stay with the individual for the rest of their lives. The effects can range from a mild rash through to severe 'flu like symptoms. And yes, both sexes can be allergic to rubber. Rubber is a natural substance which is treated with various chemicals when it's made. It's usually a reaction to these chemicals which causes the allergy, but not always. Condoms are also covered in a lubricant and spermicide and some people are allergic to these chemicals. There are 'allergy free' condoms on the market but you may have to hunt around for them.

Some people have an allergic reaction to their partners! It's not really an allergy as such - more of a mental phobia about their partner touching them in a sexual way! Women especially can have a phobia about semen going inside them - it's as though the sperm can be seen wiggling around that terrifies them. And in men, usually younger men, the thought of making any sexual contact with their partner can produce a nervous rash coupled with a feeling of nausea.

Counselling can help with these phobias but with an understanding and perhaps frustrated partner, the problem can often resolve itself.

64. Why so some young people have so many sexual partners?

I assume we're talking about boy/girl relationships here? Yes, some are friskier than others and there are three main reasons: one, that younger people tend to have a greater sex drive and sex is so enjoyable that they want to try or 'experiment' with as many people as possible. Two, that sex is a great urge like hunger and they don't always find things so appetising on the first and further encounters, and constantly try to find satisfaction and compatibility elsewhere. And third younger people tend

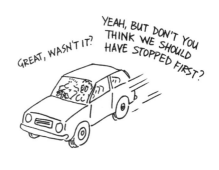

GREAT, WASN'T IT?

YEAH, BUT DON'T YOU THINK WE SHOULD HAVE STOPPED FIRST?

to get a kick out of doing something new that makes them feel independent of their parents or those adults that are around them. Sex becomes a form of escape and each new contact becomes an adventure, exciting and morale-boosting.

So all the time there's innate sexual curiosity and the sexual drive to accompany it, permissiveness will continue.

65. Why do men produce so many sperms?

200-300 million do seem a little over generous - but then, who's counting? Do you realise that 250 million is about the population of America and only one lucky sperm is going to pass on its DNA code? About 25 percent of all sperm are abnormal. Some have two heads or large heads with no tails, some have small heads with too much tail while others are so deformed, they look curly like pubic hair!

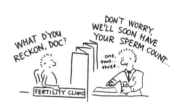

Then, 60 percent run out of the vagina virtually straight after intercourse. Those that remain high up in the cervical mucus are suspended and the natural acidity kills off a load more. Some get really frightened and can't swim too well, but one in 2000 do manage to find their way up into the womb. It's dark and horrible in there and not a nice place to spend a Saturday night. Some more get killed off or run out of energy. Then they have to find their way into one of the two Fallopian tubes where, hopefully, an egg is waiting. Even when they do meet an egg - a real giant compared with their size, how do they know what to do? Perhaps 250 million isn't enough!

66. I understand that too many sexual partners can lead to cervical cancer. Why is this?

Too many sexual partners can lead to a lot of things! The cervix is the neck of the womb and yes, it is at special risk from sexually transmitted infections. One infection in particular, the human papilloma virus, which causes genital warts, is found in many cases of cervical cancer. So, doctors fear that this virus 'triggers off' the cancer.

Women who start having sexual intercourse at an early age, as well as those who are sexually promiscuous have a higher risk of the cancer developing - or at least a cervical pre-malignant condition. It's always sensible for women to have a regular cervical smear.

Worldwide, cervical cancer is the second most common cancer in women, with a much higher incidence in the Western world. Women under 25 years rarely contract cervical cancer but the occurance in women under 35 is increasing.

The use of condoms can help prevent this condition and really it's up to all women to be more vigilant.

According to a well known magazine the largest human penis recorded was that belonging to a most unfortunate African. He was afflicted by elephantitis of the penis. It was two and a half feet long and four feet in diameter. It weighed more than 70 lbs (32kgs). Amputation seemed the only cure and, indeed, that's what happened.

67. I've been married a long time. How can I teach my husband to be more romantic?

Firstly, your husband may not realise that he's unromantic - he may think that you are! He may be simply reacting to your negative attitude. Are you sure you're making the best of yourself... would you fancy you, if you were your husband!?

A lot of women do complain about their husbands not being romantic after so many years of marriage. They also complain that they're not affectionate and these feelings - or lack of them, spill over into their sex lives and can lead to feelings of inferiority, complete lack of self-esteem and eventually, depression. It can 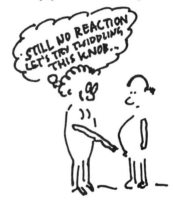 be a downward spiral and all the time, the husband is unaware that he is mainly the cause.

Men can regard romance as being effeminate or as a ploy to encourage sexual activity - especially early on in a relationship. Romance and older men are not usually compatible!

Communication is probably they key. Reward him in very subtle ways and give him praise at even the slightest polite or romantic things he might do or say. In other words, you will have to coax him along. You mustn't give up.

It's rather like having an old engine that won't go. It used to, years ago. You can't expect it to suddenly rip into life. It takes a lot of hard work to adjust all the bits and pieces. Then once it does start up, it'll need a lot of knob-twiddling to ensure smooth running. It will be a constant labour of love and the fine-tuning will be your responsibility. Only you will be able to ascertain whether it'll be all worth it!

Did you know: Most of today's sexual averages and responses, including some of those mentioned in this book, have been obtained from the research carried out by Masters and Johnson in 1960 - 65. They took 382 anonymous men and 312 anonymous women and watched what they did under laboratory conditions!

Did you know: In the 16th Century when syphilis was wide spread in Europe, the British called it the French disease, the French called it the Italian disease and the Italians called it the Spanish disease. The Japanese called it 'manka bassam' - the Portugese disease.

Did you know: Human sperm counts are almost three times those of a gorilla.

Did you know: In Roman times, the worst insult you could bestow on a woman was to accuse her of having a long clitoris.

68. Why do some people use whips and spank each other?

Couples do all sorts of things to one another when they become sexually excited because..er...er...they like to! All's fair in love and sex! Algolagnia is the clinical name of s/m or sado-masochism - the pleasure derived from giving or receiving pain. Whipping, spanking, tying up, tying down, chaining, beating and thrashing the living daylights out of one's partner can be all part of sexual activity. Drugs and alcohol can also play a big part in the proceedings and a good time is had by one and all! (Providing the neighbours don't hear).

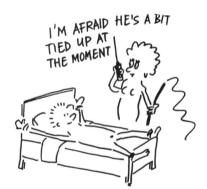

I'M AFRAID HE'S A BIT TIED UP AT THE MOMENT

According to Dr K Rix,a clinical psychologist, sado-masochism falls into two categories. First, there are those who inflict pain for sexual kicks and know what they're doing and know when to stop and second, there are those who carry on without regard or respect for the feelings of others. There is a huge difference between 'sex play' and out-and-out cruelty.

69. My boyfriend says he sometimes has a slight pain on orgasm. What do you think is wrong?

Have you remembered to remove your underwear when making love? Some young men get so carried away, they tend to overlook the obvious! A pain in the penis is rare. Your boyfriend should go and see his doctor and explain the exact type of pain he's experiencing and tell him where it seems to be coming from.

It could be a local infection, a bladder infection, a urinary tract infection or some kind of testicular disease - of which there are many. If he refuses to go, drag him along!

In some young men who are anxious and inexperienced in sexual intercourse, there is a condition called erotic orchialgia! The man gets so excited on intense sexual arousal that his whole pelvic region goes into a kind of spasm and 'locks up'. The lower pelvic muscles become tight - like a kind of cramp and this makes penetration difficult. Are you sure he's not describing these kind of pains? If it is erotica ochialgia, he must try and relax more and take his time. Sexual intercourse is so exciting for some young men that they may tend to rush things - as though they might never get another chance.

Did you know: One in ten British brides is pregnant.

Did you know: Only whales and dogs have a bone in the penis.

Did you know: The Kwakiutl Indians do not kiss each other; they suck tongues.

---

70. My older brother says he's going out with a nymphomaniac. What's he talking about?

Every young man has gone out with at least one 'nymphomaniac' in their lives. Some seem to know at least half a dozen all living in the same street! Most adolescent men have really furtive imaginations when it comes to the opposite sex. Virtually overnight, girls become a sexual conquest, a challenge to their egos - a prize to show off to their mates to show that they're real men and not boys any longer.

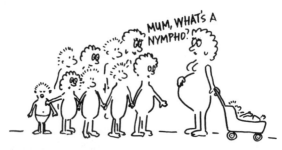

MUM, WHAT'S A NYMPHO?

Sometimes, to the guy's amazement, the girl responds. She's sexually explicit. And sexually demanding. He becomes gob smacked. Bewildered beyond his wildest dreams - the trouble is, he can't seem to handle the situation. Any sign of the least affection and she's all over him like a rash. He decides to back off a bit which could only make things worse because she tries even harder to win his failing love He dosen't know what to do: he's never been in this situation before. No one's told him that some girls have such potent sex drives and some sex drives can be very hair raising to say the least!

The only way he can resolve this predicament is to pass the blame on to the girl. He cannot be at fault. His macho image won't allow it. It has to be his partner, she's sex mad. A raving nympho! So what your brother is really saying is that he's got himself entangled with a young girl's affections and he doesn't know how to handle the situation, that's all.

In 'real life', nymphomania is a rare neurotic condition in which a woman can not achieve sexual satisfaction despite being driven by an insatiable desire for sexual intercourse. She is rarely happy and the problem can lead to many other mental disorders.

Did you know: According to a General Household Survey, 30 percent of women between 16 and 49 use no form of contraception. Some are pregnant. Some are not in a relationship. Some are just not interested in sex and some are pregnant. Some are just being foolish.

Did you know: The term 'French Letter' stems from used English condoms that were washed up on South-east beaches. Local council officials blamed the French!

Did you know: The average man ejaculates around 200 million sperm (two teaspoonful) on intercourse. A pig ejects around 900,000 million and thirty two litres for the blue whale!

Did you know: Some people are asexual and possess no sex drive at all.

---

71. I am only 16 and although we use condoms when making love I can't seem to relax. How can we be really sure that condoms won't let us down?

Let me reassure you, modern condoms are extremely reliable and, if used properly, they won't let you down. Making condoms is relatively easy. Cylindrical glass moulds are dipped into huge tanks of liquid latex rubber and the condom is simply rolled off once the rubber is dry. First point: glass is always used because if there are any imperfections, the glass shatters. Metal ones did tend to last longer but could easily become scratched when the condom was rolled off. This could have caused imperfections in the rubber surface making tears more likely to occur. Second point: samples from each batch are tested to destruction at random. If there are any defects, the whole batch is destroyed. Manufacturers are aware that their products have to be absolutely perfect. One test involves a few condoms being filled with three litres of water or sometimes 25 litres of air and if they burst, they're all considered to be substandard. A condom stretched to those limits would accommodate a dinosaur's dick!

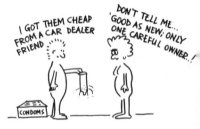

Third point: most condoms are coated in a special spermicide which kills off any sperm which might happen to creep from the base of the condom. Also most spermicides kill off bacteria and viruses that could cause HIV, herpes, gonorrhoea and other STDs so they're good at preventing infection. Fourth point: rubber is a natural substance which can stretch out of all proportion to its natural state. Fifth point: most condom factories are isolated form the outside environment to prevent dust particles entering the latex rubber solution, so preventing imperfections from occurring. Sixth point: condom factories are regularly inspected and electrical tests are carried out on the rubber to ensure no holes are permissable.

Most countries have stringent regulations about condom manufacture and in Britain, the British Standards Institute issues a 'kite-mark' seal to notify an extremely high quality of manufacture and control. Seventh point: most condoms are coated in a special lubricant to help penetration. (Sometimes, the women is not sufficiently aroused and some men are just too keen! Vaginal dryness can cause the condom to stick to the sides of the vagina and come off by a over-hasty penis).

So, the condom won't let you down but you might let yourself down by your partner not rolling on the condom early enough. It's no good stopping half way through and then remembering to take precautions. That's like trying to stop an express train at full speed. Also remember most condoms are packed in threes for a reason!

72 Why do some men 'fire blanks'?

'Firing blanks' is the cruel way of saying that a man is infertile and unable to father a child. There are many reasons for this and infertility is no way connected to a man's virility, masculinity or performance as a lover!

Up until fairly recently, male infertility was untreatable and caused so much distress that some men even committed suicide. Such was

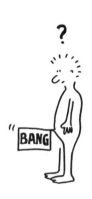

the stress put upon them to carry on the family line - to produce a son. Other similar pressures from partners, friends and close relations have had severe psychological effects on many men. There has always been a stigma attached to male infertility and consequently, many men are reluctant to be investigated for this problem.

Let's consider the main reasons for male infertility. Being overweight. Although many obese men are fertile, infertility increases with weight gain. Smoking can affect sperm count especially if sperm are being produced at a reduced number...smoking will aggravate the situation. Alcohol can cause cell damage and reduce sperm manufacture in the testes.

Drugs can also reduce sperm count. These could include 'social' drugs such as marijuana and medicinal drugs, such as antidepressants, anti malarial, blood pressure and cytotoxic drugs treating blood disorders. Excessive exercise can be a temporary cause due to a man being underweight. Stress is always a problem. It's the curse of today's living and can affect men in different ways. It does cause a reduction in sperm count but no one really knows why.

Some couples believe that too much sexual intercourse makes a man's sperm less 'volatile' but this has yet to be proven. In fact in some tests, men who have intercourse several times a day(!) are still fertile. Sometimes a woman can produce anti-bodies to her partner's sperm. Her body thinks sperm are an intrusion - like an infection and wants to eliminate them! Some men do have infected sperm and bacterial micro-organisms can be carried on their outer surfaces.

Occasionally, there are rare chromosomal defects which produce abnormal sperm or sometimes the testes don't produce any sperm at all. Five percent of infertile men have a problem called azoospermia. Some men are born without the tubes (the vas deferens) which run up from the testicle to the prostate gland. There may be blockages in these tubes or defects in the ejaculatory muscles. A severe case of mumps in childhood can affect the blood supply to the testes. There may be hormonal problems - the pituitary gland doesn't produce enough chemical signals for the testes to be stimulated.

Tuberculosis, a sporting injury or strain, or a STD may be the cause. In 90 percent of all cases of male infertility, semen with few sperm or sperm of poor quality are the cause.

73. I am 16 and my boyfriend and I tried to have sex but his penis just wouldn't go in far enough! In the end we gave up. What do you think caused my vagina to 'close tight'?

You've been trying too hard! This is a very common problem especially when young couples start fumbling their way around each other's bodies. Both parties don't really know what to expect.

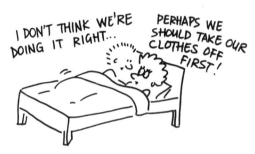

I DON'T THINK WE'RE DOING IT RIGHT...

PERHAPS WE SHOULD TAKE OUR CLOTHES OFF FIRST!

Everyone including the media make sex sound so easy - like blowing one's nose, but some first time sexual encounters can be fraught with disappointments.

Many couples who begin to have sexual relationships are unrealistic. They tend to rush the whole sex thing, and more often than not, the young man becomes far too eager and loses control right at the crucial moment! Doubts and feelings of inadequacy make the situation worse and, in your case, involuntary tightening of the strong vaginal muscles occur. Everything has a name and this problem is called vaginismus - which doesn't sound very sexy or romantic but it's one we're stuck with.

The vaginal muscles clamp together so tightly that vaginal penetration becomes impossible. The man can have a really bruised dick and possible pelvic tension resulting in muscle cramp. No matter what he does, he's unable to venture further than a few centimetres!

Other factors can also cause vaginisimus like insufficient stimulation, sexual phobias, worries about becoming pregnant, unpleasant incidenies resulting from rape or childhood sexual abuse and previous painful unpleasant sexual intercourse.

Some young women are told that sex is dirty and this can lead to muscle spasms which seem to be out of control of the woman. Choice of location can also play a part.

Some women complain of painful intercourse called dyspareunia. This can accompany vaginismus and occurs when insufficient vaginal lubricating fluid is present. The penis rubs the sides of the vagina and causes a sore burning feeling... for the man as well as for the woman! But your problem will probably go away when you and your partner become more experienced: take your time, relax and try to add an element of fun to your love-making so the whole sex act becomes more enjoyable.

74. Why are we all obsessed with sex? Men are supposed to think of sex every seven minutes of every waking hour. Why? Do you think the average hedgehog has the same sexual urges?

Their are some men who think of sex every seven <u>seconds</u> - even in their sleep!

The basic reason why humans are so obsessed with sex is that we're not very fertile and when we need to mate to pass on our respective genes. The average female animal conceives on the first 'encounter'. In Western Europe, even with the woman at her most fertile time of the month, conception is very low - the lowest it's been for 200 years. The conception rate varies with age but, when fertile partners are 25 - 30 years old, the chances of having a baby, on a single act of intercourse, is only one in three or four. (And, one in eight couples experience problems in becoming parents - and, unfortunately, one in six couples are never able to have children).

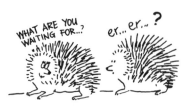

Maybe that's one of the reasons why the human penis is relatively long: it tries to deposit semen as near as possible to the opening of the womb for egg fertilisation. Even with women being able - in theory - to conceive so readily, we still need to be 'at it' more times than animals in order to reproduce.

Animals don't usually think about sex as much as humans. Food and shelter are perhaps of more importance, together with defending a territory or warding off potential rival males. (Hedgehogs are probably the exception... they probably think about it all the time, but are a little confused). Most humans have food and shelter etc. and therefore our minds are more susceptible to sexual images that we see all around us - such as on TV or in magazines, so a perceived opportunity to fantasise/to mate is always there. Our so-called higher intelligence, better health, nutrition etc, have simply enabled us to last longer than we should and so populate the world.

Did you know: In a recent American study, married men scored higher on a measure of mental health than unmarried men, while unmarried women scored higher than married women. (You can draw your own conclusions to these facts...).

Did you know: One in ten children in Britain do not have the father they think they have.

Did you know: The favourite colour for condoms in Sweden is black. In Kenya white ones are preferred.

Did you know: All men have a larger left testicle.

Did you know: There is a divorce case on record which cites unreasonable behaviour in which the husband demanded sexual intercourse after every meal.

---

75. Why do some men dress up as women?

Joan Rivers once said, 'Marry a transvestite and you double your wardrobe!' In Britain, men dressing up as women or women dressing in men's clothes are as equally common. The correct name for this practice is 'eonism' but such people are usually known as transvestites , transsexuals, cross-dressers or trannies.

Transsexuals are not mentally disturbed in a true psychological sense and may lead 'normal' lives; holding down ordinary jobs and even being married with family ties. They are usually quite happy, strong minded individuals but feel they've been born the wrong sex. It's as though their sexuality has been mixed up but they are still mainly heterosexual.

DAD, DON'T YOU FEEL A BIT OF A TIT DRESSED LIKE THAT?

Men dress up as women in order to express the feminine side of their personality and can be motivated by erotic admiration for women. The same desires occur in transsexual women but it's probably more acceptable for the average person to 'ignore' a woman who is dressed in a man's clothes. A woman dressed as a man can be regarded as an unknown quantity - a threat. However. transsexuals are very adept at disguising their true gender.

76. Do bald men really make better lovers?

This is a difficult question to answer because some men are sneaky. They wear toupees. Is a toupee-wearing man, bald? These men have a serious identity problem and any man with an identity problem is a little suspect in the sincerity stakes.

Then there are the bald men which cheat by side-combing hair which they do have. Can a man who cheats on his hair be trusted in bed? Then there are the out-an-out slapheads. Bald and proud of it. I suppose these are real men amongst baldies. They admit they're bald. No messing about. No pretence. No self-doubts. Born to be bald!

Many women don't have a choice when it comes to their partner's hair. They simply stick by them through thick hair and thin. Whether they are better lovers or not depends on how a woman treats her man and whether she accepts his loss of hair. Ultimately his ratings in the bedroom will depend on her!

Did you know: In America, a new type of contraceptive device is being developed. It's a small electrical device which is placed in the neck of the womb and emits a weak electrical current. Sperm are simply electrocuted and immobilised - suspended in cervical mucus until they die. (Sounds like a bad science-fiction movie).

Did you know: In Zimbabwe they call condoms 'little yellow raincoats'.

P.S.

Well, that's about it for this book - I'm just exhausted just thinking about sex! I'm going back home to Australia for a while.

If you'd like any questions answered, or if you have any amusing stories relating to... y'know, sex, then why not share them? You can send them to me via the Publishers.

There are still a lot of questions that have been saved up for the sequel to this book, so look out for that next year.

Thanks once again for reading "Sex Questions & Answers"...

Love

Amanda Scott

OTHER TITLES FROM IDEAS UNLIMITED (PUBLISHING)

copies "100 CHAT UP LINES"
ISBN : 1 871964 008 (128 PP A7)...................................... £1.99
copies "IDIOTS HANDBOOK OF LOVE & SEX
 ISBN: 1 871964 083 (128 PP A7)...................................... £1.99
copies "10 GOLDEN RULES OF CHATTING UP"
ISBN: 1 871964 091 (128 PP A7)....................................... £1.99
copies "SIZE ISN'T EVERYTHING"
ISBN 1 871964 121 (80 PP A7 + GIFT)........................... £1.99
copies "HOW TO WIN THE NATIONAL LOTTERY"
ISBN: 1 871964 148 (80 PP A6).. £1.99
copies "NOT WON THE LOTTERY YET THEN ?"
ISBN:1 871964156 (80 PP A6)... £1.99
copies "SEX Q & A FOR SO-CALLED EXPERTS"
ISBN: 1 871964 172 (96P A6) £1.99
copies "HAVE YOU SEEN THE NOTICE BOARD?"
ISBN: 1 871964 105 (80PP A4).. £3.99
copies "SEEN THE NEW NOTICE BOARD"
ISBN: 1 871964 180 (80pp A4).. £3.99
copies "SPORT FOR THE ELDERLY"
ISBN: 1 871964 113 (48PP A5).. £2.50
copies "BODY LANGUAGE SEX SIGNALS"
ISBN: 1 871964 067 (64PP).. £2.50
copies "THE BEGINNERS GUIDE TO KISSING"
ISBN: 1 871964 024 (64PP A5).. £2.50
copies "TIPS FOR A SUCCESSFUL MARRIAGE"
ISBN: 1 871964 032 (64PP A5).. £2.50
copies "THE JOYS OF FATHERHOOD"
ISBN 871964 040 (64PP A5)... £2.50
copies "OFFICE HANKY PANKY"
ISBN: 1 871964 059 (64PP A5).. £2.50
copies "OF COURSE I LOVE YOU"
ISBN: 1 871964 016 (96PP A6).. £1.99
copies "WELL HUNG"
ISBN: 1 871964 075 (96PP A5 Full Colour)....................... £2.99
copies "THE 9 SECONDS SEX MACHINE"
ISBN: 1 871964 164 (80 PP A7).. £1.99

I have enclosed a cheque/postal order for £.................. made payable to:

Ideas Unlimited (Publishing)

Name:...

Address:..

....

....

....

County::...................................... Post Code...................................

Fill in the coupon above and send it with your payment to:

Ideas Unlimited (Publishing)
PO Box 125
Portsmouth
Hampshire PO1 4PP

Postage free within the United Kingdom.

If you wish your purchase to be sent directly to someone else (eg: a Birthday/Christmas/Wedding/Valentines gift), simply fill in their name and address in the coupon above and enclose your cheque/postal order, with your personal message or card, if desired We will be pleased to send your gift directly to your chosen recipient..